# Baked Nuts

## The perfect recipe to make a little boy bun

By:
Dr. C. K. Blue

Copyright © 2015 B.B.R., LLC
Dr.blue.books@gmail.com

# Contents

# Preface

This book may change your life. It changed mine forever in a way I never could have imagined.

Somedays I feel worn out, exhausted, sleep deprived, nervous, anxious, and out of shape with a lack of personal identity. Then, when I least expect it, I hear this little pitter-patter coming down the hallway, getting louder as it gets closer, until a hurricane weighing in at 35 pounds dives into me, head first. His little arms wrap around my neck while he squeezes tightly for a deep, 3 second hug that wipes away all those negative emotions. I try to pause time for that brief moment of unexplainable joy, then suddenly he pulls back, looks at me with the same irresistible smile he inherited from his mother, grabs my face with his sticky hands, and tries to pick my nose. Once I prevent him from jamming his tiny finger into my sinus cavity, he jumps off me, usually tapping my royal jewels somehow with his feet, and then he takes off running.

As my stomach absorbs the pain from being kicked in the balls for the hundredth time by my son, I hear a faint cry. It's not my wife, but it's a cry of need and desire to be held. I go into her room, only to find her trying to crawl in her crib, on her hands and knees having just awakened from her afternoon nap. She hears me walk in, looks up at me while trying to control that heavy head, and gives me a huge smile.

Another recognizable smile, but not from my wife, a smile I recognize from years of looking in the mirror. She has my smile. I pick her up and she buries her head into my neck. She then pulls her head back, grabs at my beard with her sharp baby nails, and gives me another big open mouth smile.

At this point all the drama from work and the stress of dealing with everyone other than my three favorite people have disappeared. I am home. I am blessed to be home with my two children and my amazing wife. I am happy.

Our life is one big book. It begins with us in diapers, and for many, it ends with us in diapers. We are born into this world with nothing, and we leave this world with nothing. I have worked in the medical field long enough to realize one important fact of life…the fear of death disappears when your loved ones are there to hold your hand until your last breath. Life is difficult and maintaining strong relationships with your parents and children can be very trying at times, but it is worth the hard work and compromise.

This book was written to change the belief that you have no control over choosing which gender you conceive. Everyone's aunt and cousin will endorse some kind of method to have a boy or a girl. I have heard many "techniques" and some of them are so far-fetched that it seems almost impossible to replicate. You have to turn down the noise of life to see how easy it is to make a baby. We are given the basic building blocks to reproduce but the world we live in clouds our mind into thinking we have no say in the matter. There may not be 100% guarantee, but there is a way to choose a gender…naturally.

I am a doctor and I have devoted many years of my life to studying anatomy and the human body. I have been a student in gross anatomy class and I have led students through cadaver dissections. I have seen the inside and outside of countless human bodies and they have all been slightly different, but mostly the same. I have been tormented in my dreams and tested the next day about neuroanatomy and orthopedics. I have failed to comprehend, but where I struggled, I pushed harder to understand. I love the human body because it is finite and tangible, but at the same time, it is still a mystery after all these years of learning. It is truly an amazing work of art. We do not know how everything works, but it is all there, right in front of us to learn.

This book will explain how to successfully get pregnant.

This book will explain how to conceive a boy.

If you and your mate have no infertility issues or major health concerns, be careful following the two recipes in this book because you will conceive a child. And if you want a boy, the recipe in this book will produce a boy. For those who already have a boy and want a sweet little girl, skip the boy recipe and follow the girl recipe. Either way you choose, you will not be disappointed. My wife and I followed these recipes, and we got what we wanted each time.

The only drawback to following the Dr. Blue Recipe…you may decide to stop having children after you get what you want.

# Baby Dreams

What is the perfect recipe to put a bun in the oven, and how can I choose if the batter has nuts…or not?

How do I get pregnant? More importantly, how can I choose the gender at conception?

We all want a healthy baby. That is without question. God be with those children and families with disabilities, but what if we *could* choose a gender at the moment of conception? If not ensure a gender, but tip the scales heavily towards our preference. Most will argue there is no way of choosing. Many years ago, most would argue that the Earth was flat. Can the dogmatic belief of having no control over your child's sex be challenged? It all boils down to understanding two basic concepts: anatomy and gravity.

Some of the most brilliant people on Earth will say the best way to achieve greatness is to keep it simple. It is our human nature to over-think complex questions and hypothesize why and how. We are problem solvers and we like to prove theory with concrete answers. In our pursuits to explain the universe around us, we tend to overlook the essential details of life and aim higher. We feel that if we can answer the bigger problems, the rest will fall into place. This may temporarily quench the thirst for knowledge, but the fundamental life challenge will continuously surface. We have utilized our knowledge of science to overcome some of life's tallest hurdles, but we have yet to solidify a permanent answer to the question of life. We know how it all works, but we roll the dice each time we make love, praying for a yes or no in the following weeks.

Within hours after intercourse, you may have a tiny seed growing inside you, but you will not know if a boy or girl seed was planted for many weeks. Many have prayed over this question until their hands blister, begging for an answer, hoping for a gender, and wondering if they may really have to pay for another wedding one day. It may be easier for the wrong couple, and it may be difficult for the right couple, but you can make it happen if you learn the proper recipe.

Getting a positive pregnancy test will change your life. Many couples will try for years without success, while for others it seems effortless, almost unstoppable. Some will pay any price to have offspring and some will give away their children, whether it is the inability to care for them or just plain drug induced apathy. Some couples will turn to science. Others may turn to old wives tales. A child is unable to choose the life in which they are born, so before you chase the dream of having a child, make sure you understand the amount of work it takes to achieve that dream.

Some dreams are not returnable. And some dreams are worth the hard work.

What do you want most out of life? Do you want to live for yourself or do you want to live for your children? As we grow through life's stages – learn, pursue, fail, succeed – we learn lessons along the way. We strive for the dreams that we believe will bring us happiness. Then, on that glorious day when we finally touch the star that seemed so far away, we may realize it is more than a sparkly spot in the sky. In the early weeks of supporting a new life, the dream of having a baby may not be as bright as we expected. But with the hard work and sleepless nights, we find ourselves inseparable from our new found glory. With all the background noise in our daily life, it is difficult to hear the peaceful music - the simple dream - the one thing that will bring us happiness until we close our eyes for the last time… the gift of a child's unconditional love.

Continue this journey with caution. After reading this book, the dream of making a baby may be within reach. Raising a family is no easy task and it takes both a man and a woman to make a child. Children need a male *and* a female influence in their life. Before you decide to bring a baby into this world, make sure you can work together with your partner. It may be tempting to create life with many enticing mates, but before you decide to plant a seed, make sure you are attracted to their personality as well. Once you create a life, that child is going to have the same personality traits as their parents. So if you do not enjoy the company of your mate, you may have a difficult time connecting with your child.

There will be many pitfalls and snares along life's journey to finding your baby making partner in crime. Throughout life, there are traps everywhere. Ultimately, we all want to get caught in the trap, but the hardest part is finding the best trap for us…our soulmate.

If you understand the predator, you will overcome their trap. To understand how the trap works, we must start at the beginning.

# The Trap

Life is simple in the early days. As a newborn baby, we need milk from mommy's tit. It keeps us alive and makes us happy. A belly full of milk and some skin-to-skin bonding time with mommy will make anyone sleep peacefully.

As an infant, things start to get noisier. We still want mommy's tit, but now there are other things that grab our attention: lights, music, animals, and balls. Balls are awesome to infants. They are so versatile and can entertain for hours.

Just think how happy you would be right now if you had a tit in your mouth and a ball in your hands. That sums up men in one sentence. Women are way more confusing.

The toddler years lead us to believe that we want more. The doors of opportunity begin to open wide as we are convinced we want everything out there that appeals to us. Now we want two different kinds of balls. Why not three? Mommy's tit is our safe place, but we gradually venture outside our nest of comfort.

As a child, we have a short attention span, so mommy is able to pull the tit away as we soak up the world around us. The stimulation we receive from the noise of life begins to lead us into our own imaginative minds. We begin to dream big. We lose sight of where it all started.

The teenage years confuse us. We realize those childhood dreams do not sound as cool as they once were, slowly falling back to Earth from that dream of flying over the clouds. We become engulfed with media and are influenced by suggestive hints strategically placed by marketers. Adults try to warn us that people on TV are not real. We begin to learn how photo shopping and air brushing make us jealous of their "perfect" body. We believe the visual lies fed to us by models in magazines. We don't want to accept the truth that a perfect butt and six-pack abs require dedication to diet and exercise. We are young and able to crush a pint of ice cream and cookies without skipping a beat, more importantly, no extra chub in the morning.

As we continue to learn and grow from the high school years, we begin to make better decisions based on past experiences. Life becomes more complicated and the responsibilities begin to accumulate. Most of us improve our ability to think before we act. We get tired of filling the void in our life with superficial relationships and possessions.

We want fulfillment. We want happiness. We don't know what we want.

Men and woman were made to be different. We compliment each other and we need each other to survive. Women need men for all the manly things and men need women as an arbitrator for the man's two heads to work together equally. Men and women are both predators and prey, it just depends on who is chasing. Our traps are similar, but women are extremely crafty with their cleverly disguised bait.

Think about a beautiful woman in a camouflage bikini. That just confuses the hell out some men. She's obviously hunting something, and it's definitely not a deer.

We have all observed predators set traps to catch and eat their prey. The cute, furry little rabbit wanders up to the carrot. The carrot is floating in the air as if it were speaking to the rabbit.

"Come take a bite," the carrot ever so softly speaks to the rabbit.

How is that carrot majestically floating in the air? The rabbit does not care. He only sees a delicious piece of food knowing that once he eats that carrot, he will be happy. Unbeknownst to the rabbit is that the carrot comes with a price…his life! That spectacular carrot is attached to a string, and that string is attached to a baby. That baby will make or break you. You will either fold under pressure, or become a strong and wise rabbit.

If for one moment the rabbit stepped back to analyze the situation and weigh out his options, things might be different…

"Do I dare take the chance of getting the carrot before the trap is sprung? I'm fast," says the little rabbit, "I can get in and out quickly and still get a piece of carrot."

On the other hand, ponders the rabbit, "If I stick around just a bit too long, that rock will land on me and I will be taken by a predator."

Taken where? The rabbit is unsure.

Will it be a bad thing if the rock falls on the rabbit? Maybe.

Will it be a good thing? Perhaps.

"I'm a wise rabbit who has lived this long by snatching carrots. I can get some without getting caught."

Does the payoff of a delicious carrot outweigh the fear of the unknown? For most of us it does. It is that primal instinct in all of us men. We are animals and we do not learn until we try it for ourselves.

Women are smarter only because they tend to weight things out before they jump. Men, unfortunately, have two heads to persuade.

Beware of those hidden traps in bars, at gyms, and in schools. Some of the most innocent places are the most dangerous. The grocery store is filled with booby-traps, but the wise rabbit turns those traps into opportunities. The traps that are easy to spot are usually the ones to beware.

A gym is myriad of traps and snares. Beware of the ladies doing straight leg dead lifts in front of the mirror with one eye on them self and the other eye scanning for interested prey. Another obvious, but inviting trap at the gym, is the "gym clubber." This is the woman that goes to the gym with a full face of makeup, like she's just graduated from clown school, complete with big hoop earrings. She slowly rides the stair stepper, just faster than a sloth climbing a tree. She wants to get your attention by putting out the "I'm healthy and I work out vibe," however, the real truth is the junk in her trunk. Be careful not to get hypnotized by those two hams, stuffed into those tight yoga pants, steadily fighting over space to breathe. That trap says: "I don't like to exert myself and after I have kids, these two hams will explode into full bowls of cottage cheese, only to give you motion sickness if you look directly at them."

As for women, the gym is also a dangerous place of temptation. Some traps are easy to spot. The douche baggy guy that seems like he is always at the gym when you go there, doing arm curls and cable flies, wearing the tank top's cheap cousin… a t-shirt with the sleeves cut off so the nipples are just barely covered. The other guy to dodge is the one with gelled hair and trendy headphones. He's the male version of the gym clubber. They seem inviting, but they are usually shallower than a kiddie pool.

The gym can also provide lucrative opportunity. We get tired of going out to bars, battling the auction of a meat market. Some suggest going to a spin class to meet quality people, but that creates a big question in everyone's mind.

"How do I approach a woman without coming off as one of *those guys*?"

Or from a woman's perspective,

"The last thing I want is a guy trying to hit on me while I'm trying to sweat off my jiggle."

Timing is the key in that situation. It may require going to a few exercise classes before throwing some game, but it is all about a balance between humility and confidence.

Aside from a gym, college can be a plethora of pitfalls for women. Men are just trying to get a line in the water, like finding a spot on a crowded charter fishing boat. Some guys are ruthless and will take up more space. Others are not pushy because they haven't had the taste of a succulent grouper. Some guys are creepy, but most are not. Lies are abundant and inflation is even more widespread in college. The name of the game is trying to avoid stepping in too much bullshit.

Women do want to be pursued. They wouldn't be killing themselves in a spin class if they didn't want to look good naked. That is why they spend endless hours trying to master their makeup, researching the latest fashion trends and reading articles by pessimistic journalists about what men *really* want. Men are the same. They just take a different approach. They look in the mirror before walking out to the gym floor, strategically messing up their hair and checking themselves out, trying to look innocent. Men do not have the same tricks as women: push-up bras, hair extensions, and fajas.

What is a faja? Faja is spanish for lies. It makes you look skinny, but when you take it off, the body looks like a melting candle. They work, and they work extremely well! Even when men do uncover the truth, they will never turn down a naked woman. Men only wish they had something similar to hide their spare tire and man boobs.

Sadly, our society has airbrushed images into our minds of what we are *supposed* to want. The media has smothered our sense of self-confidence, but keeping an open mind can spark a romantic flame.

Not all traps are bad, and sometimes it is a good thing to be eaten alive by a sexy predator.

Just be wise and prevent yourself from becoming a remora. A remora is a sucker fish that follows a shark around the sea. The shark will never eat the remora and the remora becomes dependent on the shark, eating all their crap, day in and day out. Over time, some mates turn into remoras because their counterpart is manipulative and dominant, inconsiderate of their partner's feelings. Some of the most ruthless sharks do not live in deep water. They live on land, camouflaged by a beautiful face and a chiseled body.

Nobody deserves to be a sucker fish.

At the end of the day, most of us want to get caught in a trap. We get tired of fishing around the same pond and we dream about what else is out there. We want the next step of our life and we want to move on from the single scene. We get tired of cleaning all the bullshit off our shoes and we look over the fence to the greener, bullshitless grass.

In time, our hunting partners retire and we find ourselves hunting alone. What was once a solid wolf pack of single ladies or strapping young men has turned into a lone predator, scarred by years of poor choices and chicanery by treacherous rat snakes. Those long nights of optimistic drinking and hanging out in smoky bars, looking for "the one," will eventually lead to wrinkles and sore feet.

Pace yourself, for your body, for your mind, and for your sanity. One day you will find the one who makes you happy. Be patient and be wise because real life is full of clichés and one day lady luck will smile upon you and introduce you to someone special. The key is to be free when that person knocks on your door. If you are currently stuck in a trap, knowing in your heart that you don't want to be eaten by that predator for the rest of your life, get out now!

So you must think quickly when you find yourself in the same predicament as the little rabbit. Be wise before you spring the trap. Carefully get to know the trap before you dive in head first screaming GERONIMO as you place your dough deep into the oven. When you put a bun in the oven, you will create a mixture of the good and the not so good from both of you. Make sure your heart and soul absolutely love every inch of your partner. Your child needs both of you present to feel complete. If one bails, and no one steps in to take their place, they may become one of the traps to avoid.

# Preheating the Oven

Life is filled with traps. We understand this concept and yet we still jump head first into the trap that hypnotizes our subconscious. A vagina: full of mystery for a young man and the power it exudes is intriguing to a young woman. After a young man's first encounter with a clean escape, it only magnifies the power and draws him in for more. There is technique to the escape. On the flip side, there is technique to harnessing the power and creating something amazing...LIFE.

We have made tremendous leaps and bounds over the knowledge bridge to understanding our bodies, but we will never fully understand how all the pieces of the puzzle fit together to create such an amazing work of art. The vagina lips are the gates of life and once you witness your own child thrust into this world, head first, it will change the way you see everything!

We make bold attempts to understand physiology and explain how DNA actually works. One day we will be able to alter a baby's DNA to "prevent" adverse medical conditions. One day we will be able to choose what eye and hair color our baby sees in the mirror each day. One day may never come, but one day may come too soon.

Life will always find a way. Mutations in genes and adaptations to human intervention will follow that "one day" and life will continue to flourish in spontaneous ways. The human body is absolutely incredible and we will never be able to fully understand how all the cards fall into place. Think about all the food that we eat and all the toxins that go into our body. Somehow, our incredible machines are able to sift through all that garbage to find the correct building blocks to make a beating heart, an intricate vascular network, and a complex structural support system that is all electrically hardwired to be run manually and on autopilot. The answer to the human puzzle lies within the most amazing specimen on this planet. Men are a close runner up as the second best, but women are by far number one. Women have all the power in the world, but to get to it, you have to go through the boss.

If you want to harness the power of the life, you must first make friends with the boss.

All bosses are different. Some are a pleasure to entertain while others may be a little high maintenance. Beware the trap and remember that each boss may be around for awhile, so make sure you can mingle with the boss. As for women, take care of the boss and keep her looking good. She's important. She's the boss but she knows she has competition. She is not the only one with this power; there are many others like her.

A great relationship between the boss and the penis depends on trust and communication. To wake the boss, you must increase the circulation throughout the entire body. The boss will not be happy if you try to beat down the office door without   introducing yourself to the rest of the staff. You must stimulate the entire mind and body to get up the chain of command. Without properly exploring all the channels of the body's sensory tracks, the flow of energy may not fully be directed to the little man in the boat (we'll get to know him later). The world around us explains our body and we have to allow our mind to understand. Imagine a river: if there is no current, the water is murky; if there is a current, the water is full of fish.

To understand how sensation in the body works, a homunculus is a good visual representation. A homunculus is a figure depicting the amount of space each body part occupies in the brain. It was first popularized many years ago by a group of "scientists" to explain how the brain works. It still has some value today as a good visual image of the significance of each body part in the brain, but it is by no means the full story. The power of touch is extremely valuable if applied properly, but some other areas on the homunculus need to be enlarged. The point is that the hands, tongue, and lips are among the biggest portions, which may be accurate, but the homunculus was developed many years ago and needs some revision. One of the areas was not given enough credit.

The tongue is similar to the hammer. It is one of the oldest tools in the shed and a man with a hammer can fix anything. Directions on how to use the hammer will be reviewed shortly. It takes more finesse than just hammering the boss as hard as possible. You have to use all the tools in your tool box if you want to make the perfect bun. Save the hammer, pull out the power tools first... use the hands.

Hands are extremely powerful tools, but they are not as straight forward as the tongue. The power of skin to skin touch is undeniable. There are millions of neural receptors in the skin that stimulate physiological responses from the rest of the body. A baby in the neonatal intensive care unit can make miraculous improvements while lying naked on a bare skin chest. An adult can be pulled from a pit of depression with just a simple, deep hug. An elderly man or woman can improve their will-power with the touch of a small child. Although it may be difficult to scientifically explain why and how, the power of touch is real.

With a simple stroke of the hand, a man can make a woman tremble with goose bumps. With a gentle touch, a woman can persuade a man to do whatever she desires. It is all in the touch. If you have ever played a sport, a musical instrument, or crafted art, you may realize how different an outcome may be with just the right touch.

So how do you preheat a woman's oven just by touch…with your heart and inner strength.

The skin is one large organ that separates us from the outside world. It enables us to keep it all together, literally. It is full of receptors that pick up different stimulations and transmit the chemical responses to our brain. How we interpret those stimulations and how we respond are a combination of learned behavior and primal instinct. A familiar smell is a powerful way to trigger a memory, like smelling a delicious food can trigger hunger. Just the right touch can trigger a response of hormones that will flood the brain with a pleasurable interpretation. Finding just the right touch depends on who you are touching. Not all animals respond the same.

We will review the most important staff members of the body to meet before you go to the boss, but first you must learn to let go of the world around you. Focus all of your energy into your hands. This is where the inner strength comes into play. It is a difficult aspect of the human body to quantify, but there is energy that flows through our bodies. Many different practices like yoga, martial arts, and mediation teach people how to focus the energy within and transfer it through their body to a specific destination. With practice you may feel a wave of energy throughout your body. You can find many resources to assist in developing your focus of inner strength, but we are not breaking bricks. We are turning our sexual partner's oven on broil so we can put a bun in that nice hot oven. Remember, it is not only important to preheat the oven, it is also important for the man to get those seeds ready for launch when the right moment happens.

For a man to successfully make a bun with nuts, he must learn how to transfer his energy from his hands, to his tongue, and then out through his penis.

A light touch is all it takes. A slow, delicate stroke down the side of her face, the inside of her elbow, the outline of her side breast and along the ribs can begin the process. Gently glide your finger tips across the contours of her body to stimulate the skin and hair follicles along a continuous path. You can gently graze by the nipples, but keep your partner guessing where you go, hoping you while find your way to the boss, but wondering what you will do next. The element of surprise heightens the emotions and stimulates the hormones to unload throughout the body. Use your hands and your lips, gently kissing every area of the body, periodically catching eye contact, but not too much eye contact to cause feelings of insecurity.

The last thing you want in this moment is for your partner to question their confidence of their body or their feelings.

For the man to successfully stimulate the flow of energy throughout her body, he must gently explore the entire female canvas, eventually bringing his hands back together, with each hand on one side of the body, sliding down the sides of the breasts, stopping at the nipples for a quick hello, and down around the pelvis to the pubic shelf. Do not go below the pubic shelf. Not yet. This is the bone just above the genitals. Think of it as a finish line to meet the boss. Instead, go south along the inside of the thighs to the feet or gently slide your hands up the front of the torso; this time along the inside of the breasts, back up to the side of her face and into her hair. Most women like their hair pulled to some degree. The amount of pressure depends on the woman but grabbing at the roots and applying a gentle pull will continue to heat that oven. If you decide to go south to the feet, massage the soles of her feet and her heels with a light stretch of the achilles and separation of the foot bones.

Do not stay at the southern most point too long. If a foot rub is in order, begin down there and work your way up, otherwise, stay focused and keep your eye on the prize. We're making a bun...maybe two.

For a quick tip on preheating the oven, an ankle massage is the perfect time to let the tip of the penis graze along her vagina lips. Ladies, give him a hand to direct his penis along the contours of the vagina, but do not allow the penis inside the boss's office. Stay out. You can poke your head inside to let her know you are waiting outside, but do not go all the way in, just the tip.

As you work your way north, kiss her inner thighs and wrap your hands around the outside of her hips. Apply some manly pressure to let her know you are about to ravage her, but don't go overboard, be gentle. Skip right on by the boss and work your way back up the torso, kissing along the inside of her breasts, sliding your hands along the inside of her upper arms, interlocking each other's fingers as you sink in for a deep kiss.

At this point, she should be feeling very anxious, and he should too. He must make an attempt to touch and kiss almost every inch of her body…almost every inch. There are a few square centimeters of real estate you should not kiss on a woman. Keep in mind you are trying to prepare yourself for the right moment. The man's preparation is just as important as preheating the woman's oven. Timing cannot be emphasized enough. Visualize everything you want to do to her. Go over the next 20 minutes in your head so you are ready to orgasm when the time is right. As the man, you are in control, and you must make sure you both orgasm at the same time. If you need some help, now is the time. Guide her hands and even her lips if necessary, but do not push her too hard, or you will open the oven door and let some of the heat out. Know your partner. Become familiar with each other's sexual buttons. Practice, practice, practice.

Her oven should be so hot that she is begging for it. The key to a successful bun is a pulsating, hot oven. Once it is hot, all it takes is a spark and some dough. All the work up to this point has been to get that oven preheated. The bun is not ready to go in the oven just yet.

# The Little Man in the Boat

Life is all about relationships. In order to have a successful relationship with the boss, you must first become best friends with the little man in the boat. But who is this little man in the boat and does he really have magical powers?

Life as an adolescent in America does not seem unique, however, when we were that age, most of us would disagree. Middle school was a wild jungle and its close proximity to the high school years lead many youth to the extremes of prosperity or persecution. Some of the quickest events in our lives molded our perception of the world around us. What some adults perceive as a minor verbal chat with a youth may have a lasting effect on that child's view of life.

The 90's were just the beginning of the internet, so we did not have access to all of life's questions on a phone, tucked away in our pocket. If we had a question about sex, we could only speculate as to what it really meant while gossiping around a lunch table until the topic somehow got us into trouble. Sex education class for boys was an hour or two of trying not to laugh every time the teacher said penis or vagina. I can only imagine how awkward it was for the girl's class. It must have been extremely terrifying to actually see a live birth on a VHS tape or laser disc.

As we grow, we learn. And as we learn, we continue to grow. This brings us back to the trap. Once we learn more about those traps, we become intrigued and we want to learn more, seeking out more and searching for the next big experience. Learning about sex can be embarrassing and uncomfortable at times.

There was a girl in my seventh grade class who crazy about me. She had all the confidence in the world and she did not hold back her feelings towards me. Other boys in my class were jealous that she liked me, which caused them to dislike me, and I was so shy that I didn't know how to respond to her advances. She made it very clear what she wanted to do to me and I was terrified because I wasn't sure what it meant.

My parents were great about educating me on the birds and the bees, but it was still uncomfortable talking to my dad about sex. On the way to football practice, we had "the talk." After he was done explaining, he asked if I had any questions. I sat there next to him in the single cab pickup truck and thought silently for a few minutes. Then finally I had to ask. It was something that a lot of boys were talking about at school and I thought I knew what it was but I wasn't sure. It was something that girl had said to me that made me nervous.

I turned to my dad and said, "What's a blow job?" My dad was slightly taken back, trying to swallow a laugh as he quickly cleared his throat. He then casually explained to me that it was pretty much the opposite of what it sounds like.

Once my dad finished his uncomfortable explanation of a blow job, I was even more terrified. For the next two hours at football practice, all I could think about was that girl and what she said to me. Why did she want to do that to me? I knew I wanted to experience that, but I was extremely nervous. What if I did something wrong? What if every other girl at school found out and ruined it for me…forever? It was that feeling you get when you are standing at the edge of a cliff, about to jump into the water, knowing everyone else before you landed safely, but still, you are afraid to jump.

The reason why that girl left a lasting memory from my young life was not because of what she wanted to do to me, but what I learned about her from my uncle.

My mom's little brother was about 38 years old going on 17. He had just been released from prison for driving on a suspended license and was living on my top bunk until going into rehab for substance abuse. I had no fear about him sleeping above me for 30 days. He is still a great guy; he just has some demons that he can't shake. Regardless, he had a thorough knowledge of *everything*, especially females! In my mind he had pretty good credibility since he had five kids. He did hold back at times. I would ask him something and I could tell that he was trying to tame it down for 13 year old ears. I'm sure my mom put the fear of God in him not to ruin my childhood innocence, and the fact that my father was 6 foot 3, 240 pounds of solid steel made him tread lightly in our house.

He was the first person ever to mention the little man in the boat. Little did I know he would change my life forever.

One day the girl who was chasing me called our house. My uncle answered, and of course, embarrassed me when he realized a girl was calling to flirt with me. Creepily, but innocently, he began to flirt with her in a non-threatening way in an attempt to make me look good. I'll never forget what he told me after he handed me the phone….

"Don't be afraid of the little man in the boat," as he looked at me with a huge grin.

I laughed uncomfortably, but had no idea what he meant. I picked up the phone and she was laughing. She repeated it like she knew exactly what he meant, but something told me she had no idea either. Nonetheless, I let it go at the time. I would periodically ponder about what he said, but I never had the guts to ask. This was before I had a computer, and there was nothing about *some little man and his boat* in the Encyclopedia Britannica sitting on our bookshelf, collecting dust since the 80's.

The question plagued me for years until I finally identified this mystery man. He is not some fictional, mythological person. He is real and he is the most important man in the world. He is the gatekeeper. He is the doorman and the bouncer. He is the one man you want to impress in order to have a successful meeting with the boss. He is the man that will forever change your life if you rub him the right way. Most importantly, he is the key puzzle piece to putting a bun in the oven.

The little man in the boat is the clitoris.

This small piece of anatomy plays a vital role in continuing the human race. It may be overlooked by many men; however, some men understand the true power. The boss (aka the vagina) is only the face of the business. The clitoris is actually the brains behind the whole operation. Proper stimulation of the little man will open a flood gate of hormones and fluids designed to enhance the delivery of the sperms. The process of making the little man happy is not difficult. It is all about technique and perseverance.

When referring back to the homunculus, I said earlier that it needs some revisions, mainly the genitals. Anatomy can be a tricky thing to conceptualize, but once you see human anatomy, it is easily digestible. Men's anatomy is on the surface and is visible. Women's anatomy is under the surface and can be confusing. The clitoris is basically a miniature penis. The part that is visible is only the glands of the clitoris, just like the penis head. Underneath the surface of a woman is the rest of the iceberg, the crura of the clitoris. The crura are legs that split off onto each side of the vaginal canal. Think of a penis, shrink it down and butterfly it down the middle, then pull it internally so that just the head is visible. Now you have a highly innervated pleasure button, attached to many different surrounding nerves.

There are seven different major nerves that are involved in a woman's orgasm. There are only two nerves that flex the elbow, enabling us to feed our self. You pick which is more important.

Think of the clitoris as the spark plug to make the oven explode.

Biologists will support the concept that a spark of energy at the right time and in the right place can create life. By preheating the oven to the right temperature, we create an environment for life to begin. Add in a bolt of lightning from the little man and you have a perfect environment to bake a delicious bun. You need a lightning strike in order to create a baby.

# *FOUR!!!!*

Life flourishes from stimulation. If you add the proper stimulation, you will achieve your goal. The difficult part is determining the correct goal.

In the past, there was no conclusive evidence to support the need for a woman's orgasm. Most supported the idea that the orgasm was solely for pleasure. It was thought that the only reason for a female orgasm was to keep her coming back for more. Modern research has concluded otherwise. If we were to examine every inch of a human body, we would be able to identify a reason for each piece of anatomy. Our bodies are extremely intelligent designs and everything has a purpose. To think that the only reason for a clitoris and the female orgasm is pleasure would be undermining the complexity of a work of art. It is not taboo to scientifically study what happens inside the most amazing creature, during her most powerful moment. A research experiment centered on clitoral stimulation may be ethically and morally challenging in a modern world, which may be the reason why it is still partially misunderstood. However, the winds are changing and the archaic thought process of the past is disappearing while new pioneers dig deep for discovery.

If you discuss a woman's orgasm with an anatomist, they will enlighten your world. Some anatomy and physiology experts support the theory that a woman should have at least 3 orgasms from oral stimulation prior to penetration. With each orgasm, fluids are released that play a vital role in transmission and prevention. These fluids lubricate the vaginal walls to prevent irritation and ease penetration. This response promotes a more pleasurable experience and protects valuable real estate. The fluids have other important roles like neutralizing urine to prevent sperm damage and decreasing the risk of spreading sexually transmitted diseases. Getting your female partner to achieve 3 orgasms before you get your penis in the game may be difficult. She may take your penis by force if not careful.

There are also many other benefits from an orgasm that go beyond creation of life. Studies support that an orgasm improves sleep, is a form of exercise, and reduces stress. It increases blood flow to the brain while releasing endorphins that reduce pain. Research suggests that an orgasm is beneficial in preventing heart disease, breast cancer, incontinence, and painful menses. An orgasm can also decrease spasticity and muscular spasms in those with cerebral palsy. The vagus nerve is one of the seven nerves involved in an orgasm and it skips the lower spinal cord, sending excitation directly to the top while affecting many other organs along the way.

There are many references as to how to properly stimulate a woman into having an orgasm. It is not difficult; it just takes a little practice.

So let's pick up from where we left that oven. Nice and hot, burning with desire and anxious for some action. This moment in the sexual encounter is a crucial fork in the road. This is the time, as man, you must make your decision based on your track record. Are you quick to finish? Are you a master of control and can climax at command? Or does it take a while to get across the finish line?

You must remember that the point of this endeavor is to create a baby, so you want to finish quickly. If you delay too long, the oven may lose some heat and it may not work as efficiently.

If it takes you awhile to climax, go ahead and do what is necessary to get yourself close to finish. One thing to keep in mind is that you need oral stimulation on the clitoris to achieve the orgasm that will create the spark of life. Orgasm through penetration is not as effective. If you have to go in, do what you must, but make sure you grab a hand towel so you can give a quick wipe before going back downtown. Yes, you must finish her off orally, so keep that in mind. Talk it over with your partner. Make a plan if you have to. This may provide good leverage to convince her that she needs to start the game off using her head. You are trying to create a baby, so it is okay to game plan in order to get to the finish line.

So now the man is close and ready to explode, like a full glass of water about to spill. It is now time to give that little man in the boat the business. You came to see the boss, you met everyone else in the office, and now the last thing between you and the boss is the little man standing in his boat.

It is time to pull out the hammer and hammer that little guy until he submits. It's tongue time.

There is more than one way to skin a cat, and there is more than one way to stimulate a clitoris, but we are not skinning cats, so try to focus on one technique. The key to success is consistency. Stay consistent with your moves. Sometimes it is fun to get the woman close to finishing, but then back off just before she explodes. That technique is great when trying to prolong the sexual experience in order to achieve a hard orgasm, but many men have found that it may backfire if done too much. The woman may get frustrated and irritated, forcing you to put a little more heat back into the oven. So proceed with caution. But again, it is baby time, so do not delay the fun. Get your hammer (your tongue) and tickle that little man in his boat until he submits. Flicking your tongue up and down works great but some like to go in circles. You can touch on the vagina lips periodically, but stay focused on the little man hiding in his boat.

Do not get fancy. Just think of it as a light switch that you are trying to turn on and off as fast as you can with your tongue.

Maintain a constant speed and pace yourself. You may sporadically hit her with a few fast strokes to keep her guessing, but consistency is the key. Practice using your tongue muscles to build up some endurance. It may take 5 minutes, or it may take longer. The better you preheat the oven, the quicker she will get there. For the man, keep in mind what is going on so you do not lose your steam. Focusing too hard on hammering the little man can make things limp. Keep in mind what you are doing and visualize whatever is necessary to stay ready. Do not start daydreaming, unless it is about how sexy your girl is at this moment. The mind is a powerful tool of imagery; use it to keep yourself on the edge of that cliff of ejaculation.

For a woman to successfully hit the peak screaming, it is crucial to shut down her prefrontal cortex. This is the area of the brain that is constantly thinking about other non-sexual thoughts. She needs to focus on the job at hand. Use your hammer to get rid of the work day, the thoughts about bills and shopping, the daily schedule, and most importantly, the thought about getting pregnant. She needs to have a blank mind while you drop a pleasure bomb on her entire system.

The best position to achieve success is where the woman is lying on her back, with her butt near the edge of the bed. The man is at the side of the bed, on his knees. The man wants to avoid excessive neck extension in order to properly use his tongue muscles. If the man is lying on his stomach while trying to perform this act, he may fatigue quickly. It is difficult to sit with your face to the sky and flick your tongue as fast as possible, so position yourself properly. Also, the man is able to control the environment better while he is on the floor. The woman can rest her legs on the man's shoulders or place them on his thigh if he is on one knee. Many women have some form of scoliosis, so finding a comfortable spot is important. Try to avoid placing the woman's legs in a dependent position, meaning, don't make her use her own muscles to hold up her legs. If she does, this may take her mind off the goal at hand and slow things down tremendously.

Some sexual "experts" recommend stimulating the entire undercarriage in a circular fashion. The so called experts say that not only the clitoris, but also the vagina lips, need to be stimulated in a constant circular pattern in order to achieve climax. The idea is that by stimulating the entire package, you are stimulating the legs of the clitoris underneath the surface, thereby leading to an overall increase in neural stimulation. It does take some practice to truly understand your lover, so make time for practice.

In the bedside kneeling position, the man has better control of the woman's body and it is easier to stimulate the nipples. If done properly, you will only need your hammer for the little man in the boat, so use your hands to remind the twins that they are important too. Give the nipples their finder's fee of attention. They are a woman's fishing lures.

Remember that spontaneity during the final push for the spark is not recommended. You want consistency and constant nipple stimulation to magnify the effect. If you have the coordination, roll both nipples in opposite directions with a medium pressure. Think of it as trying to bend the nipple over to touch the areola and then roll it around like you are setting a clock hand. If you can only reach one nipple, that works too. Just try to keep it consistent at this point. Try not to stop and start excessively. Do not redirect power and attention away from the little man.

Forget about the "G-spot." This area is a small patch of land inside the vaginal canal. It is suggested to be on the front, upper vaginal wall; however, its existence has not been proven. The man who coined this term did so in the 1940's and establishing its existence has been challenging. New theory suggests that this spot only stimulates the legs of the clitoris through layers of soft tissue. Since all anatomy has variations, concrete evidence that "G-spot stimulation" promotes a female orgasm is devoid. Do not get fancy. Do not try to stick your fingers in there to find a magical spot. Hammer that little man.

You will know when she is about to climax. You should feel the surge of energy run through her body. Her legs will become tense. Her breathing pattern will become faster and shallower, periodically holding and catching her breath. She may pull you in tight with her legs and grab your hands, which should be on her nipples at this point applying a gentle squeeze.

Keep hammering!

Whatever you do, do not stop!

You will feel the rush of energy flood through her body. You want her to climax and you want her to hit that peak at full steam.

It is imperative to maintain your erection at full strength while she is about to burst. The man's big moment is quickly approaching and you do not want to play catch up; timing is critical.

As she makes that last push to the top of the mountain, there will be a brief calm before the lightning storm. Time will stop for a split second right before the surge of hormones flood through her body like a river exploding through a dam. She will go into trunk flexion, pulling her legs off the man's body and into her stomach, trying to get away from that hammer. The little man will have been beaten into submission and he will command the rest of the body to retreat. The little man tries to get the boss out of harm's way, somehow knowing that she is very vulnerable at this time.

Now is the time to strike!

Stand from the kneeling position, at the side of the bed, wrap you hands around the woman's upper thighs and pull her vagina to the edge of the bed. Slide your fully erect penis past the little man into the boss's office.

Your goal as a man is to orgasm and ejaculate as quickly as possible.

As you continue to thrust your penis in and out, use the rhythm your mate likes best. This should be learned during the practice sessions. Does she like it fast with a forceful finish, or does she like a more controlled, fluid motion with finesse. It is important for her but also for him. The woman has just orgasmed, so whatever works best to get the man to ejaculate is critical to achieve success. You need to get your seed into that vaginal canal as quickly as possible. Her cervix is pulsating from the rush of hormones during her orgasm. Now is the time to drop your seed into the trap. If you are slow to finish, then practice, practice, practice

Once you feel you have crossed that point of no return, visualize a transfer of energy from within your chest to your pelvis.

Grab her thighs. Whether she is on her back or knees, bend forward slightly, take a big deep breath, and then thrust into her while squeezing your butt and pelvic floor muscles, pushing your hips forward, letting out your entire load with a forceful exhale, screaming FOUR!!!! Contract every muscle you can feel in you pelvic region to push every last sperm out of your penis. You want to get every possible child to the back of the office to ensure a positive pregnancy test.

The oven was hot, you hammered the little man until he let out the spark of life, and now you dropped your seed into her like dumping gasoline onto a fire. The transfer of energy from your hands, to your tongue, and then out through your penis has completed. You can call it quits at this point and leave the rest up to chance if you truly have no preference on gender, or you can add some positional intervention and tip the scales one way or the other.

You have now reached one of the most pivotal forks in the road you call "my life." Do you want a boy or girl? You do have a choice…more than you think.

# Honey Bear Boy

Life is not always as complicated as it seems. There are many tales told by old wives that say you should eat this or that to improve your chances of having a boy. Some rely on whether the bull looks to the sun, and some say you should avoid drinking milk. You can track ovulation, make a calendar, and try to get pregnant at specific times during a woman's cycle. The Chinese culture has developed an entire calendar system to predict a baby's gender based on age and date of conception. Currently, there is minimal support from medical literature that endorses the ability to influence a baby's gender at conception. These are just theories, not facts. A theory is usually considered accurate until otherwise proven wrong by objective evidence. If we look at anatomy, the answers are clear. The hurdle in proving this theory is that life is spontaneous and tends to avoid guarantees.

For the woman, there are a few constants. She will either drop eggs or not. Some women are extremely fertile and some are not, but those eggs are in there and they are in the same location. Her eggs may have difficulty sticking to the uterine wall, but sooner or later, one will get stuck. The sperms, on the other hand, are not constant.

There is a wide range of variation among male sperm. They either carry a female chromosome or a male chromosome and one load may contain billions of swimmers. Some sperm are healthy while others may have two heads. Some may be strong swimmers and some may swim in circles. Simply ejaculating into a woman's vaginal canal does not necessarily mean they will go to the correct destination. If you properly orient the sperm, the healthy swimmers will find the egg. In order to direct sperm, you have to use gravitational forces. Gravity is crucial for life to exist on Earth, and without it, life would be no more.

To deny gravity's role in human reproduction is ludicrous.

After a sperm has been released from its testicular home, is will begin to swim in a semi-straight line. By directing the sperm, you not only improve your chances of getting pregnant, you can also give one gender an upper hand in reaching the finish line first.

Novel concepts are not well received in the medical community without reliable, objective measures, and this theory may be difficult to prove through a formal research design. Many will dispute this theory that you may actually have the ability to choose a baby's gender.

Consider the differences between a girl sperm and a boy sperm. A girl sperm is similar to a long distance runner: a slower pace with greater endurance. A boy sperm is more similar to a sprinter: fast out of the gates but quickly runs out of gas. Then consider the distance the sperm must travel in order to reach the finish line. If the boy sperm runs out of energy before he reaches the egg, the girl sperm may swim past him. If you assist the boy sperm by shortening the distance as much as possible, he should have enough gas in the tank to reach the egg first. There is one simple way to manipulate the distance of the sperm race…gravity!

How does gravity affect gender selection? The answer lies in the most magical place on Earth…between a woman's thighs.

Understanding a woman's anatomy is not difficult when you have anatomy textbooks and pioneers who have laid the foundational pipes of knowledge. If you look at a woman's pelvis from a sagittal view (side shot), you will easily comprehend the value of applying gravity to the equation. The orientation of a woman's vaginal canal mirrors a man's fully erect penis…an upward curve.

A man's penis was made to fit in the vaginal canal. Men have a ligament that assists the penis in curving up while erect. This positions the penis towards the cervix, the back of the vaginal canal. The sperm have to get past the cervix in order to find the egg. When a man ejaculates, he does so with enough velocity for his swimmers to reach the cervix. By applying some positional intervention, the boy swimmers will reach the finish line first.

In order to make a little bun with nuts, follow this recipe for success. The man must do all prep work, so he must read the recipe and follow the directions exactly. This is a week long effort on his part to set the mood and make this work everyday for 7 days. The woman has the difficult task of cooking the bun and delivering it into this world, but she must comply with her mate. Women are most fertile when they are ovulating, but a woman's ovulation period may fluctuate, based on hormones or even a stressful day at work. In order to truly make this successful, you need to follow this exact recipe.

The Dr. Blue Recipe for a little boy:

1.  Once the woman has finished her menstrual cycle, wait 7 days and perform the following recipe once a day for the next 7 days.

2.  Preheat the oven. Begin by deeply kissing your woman. Gently touch and kiss every square inch of her amazing body. Make sure you turn on every nerve in her entire body and shut down the world around her in order to get the oven to broil.

3.  Once her body is properly preheated. Say hello to the little man in the boat. Make sure you tickle him with your tongue in a consistent, yet rapid motion. Stimulate that little man, commonly known as the clitoris, until he lets out a bolt of lightning throughout her entire body. Do not forget to give some love to the nipples.

4. Once your woman achieves an orgasm from oral stimulation by your tongue, quickly insert your penis into of her vagina. Get yourself to the verge of ejaculation as quickly as possible, but do not let it release.

5. In the seconds prior to ejaculation, pull your hips back and take a deep breath. Now transfer the energy inspired by that deep breath from your chest down to your core and out through your penis.

6. Push your penis inside of her as deep as possible by extending your hips and squeezing your butt cheeks together. Unleash your seeds while you let out a strong exhale. Contract your abdominals and pelvic floor muscles to squeeze every sperm out of your penis.

7. **<u>THIS IS THE MOST IMPORTANT STEP</u>**. Once all of your sperm have been unloaded, quickly invert the woman by grabbing her upper thighs and lifting her into a hand stand. Hold your woman upside down for 20 - 30 seconds.

8. Lie her back down onto the bed and keep her horizontal for at least an hour. Do not let her get up for anything. She can lift her head to drink some water, but make sure

she stays lying flat. Preferably on her stomach.

9. Start thinking about baby boy names.

Imagine you are trying to get honey out of jar, but in this case, you are trying to get your man nectar as deep inside of your woman as possible. The hand stand is crucial to ensure a boy sperm gets to the egg first.

This is an easy recipe to follow but there are a few helpful tips to know beforehand. Obviously, all the prep work is extremely important. Make sure that oven is preheated to broil. Do not try to have a meeting with the boss before confronting the little man in his boat. Hammer that little man in his boat until he lets out a bolt of lightning. Use your power tools (your hands) to roll her nipples while hammering the little man. Remember that the nipples were most likely the bait for the trap, so spread the love.

Once you get that little man to tap out, get your penis in the game and try to get to the finish line as quickly as possible. The goal is to ejaculate within 30 seconds of your female's orgasm. Do not waste time. Practice is the key to success.

This is the reason why most guys are so quick to orgasm. Nature intended it to be that way.

As you reach the point of no return, pull back so that half of your penis is inside of her, take a deep breath and exhale while pushing your penis into her vagina as deep as allowed. Contract all the muscles in your abdominals, pelvis, and buttocks in an effort to push all of your energy, and sperm, out through your penis and into your mate.

During your practice sessions, train yourself how to breathe deeply and contract all those muscles simultaneously during the exhale. To understand how to contract your pelvic floor muscles, imagine you are trying to stop urinating. When you have an erection, your penis should rise up and the head should increase in size due to the increased blood flow from contracting your pelvic floor muscles. By contracting all these muscles during exhalation, you should be able to release as many swimmers as possible. Do not hurt your future baby momma, but if you want that boy, push that sperm into her as far as possible.

The man should be standing at bedside with her on the bed while he orgasms. This allows him to grab her upper thighs and pull the woman into an inverted position.

If she is on her back, wrap your arms around her thighs close to her hips and swing her body off the bed, into a hand stand. If she is face down, doggy style, or bent over, do the same by embracing her upper thighs and swinging her around into a front hand stand. Holding her close to her pelvis will enable you to control her center of mass and make it easier for you to position her properly. The seconds immediately following ejaculation are the most critical…she must be upside down for this moment.

Hold the woman's thighs while she maintains a hand stand for about 20-30 seconds. Give her some help by bear hugging her thighs and taking weight from her arms, assisting her to hold the hand stand.

After the upside down time is complete, the woman lies on the bed and rests, preferably on her stomach. Try not to get up for anything. Take a nap. Wash up in a couple hours. Whatever she does, do not let her urinate!

Allow that man honey to marinate.

By doing the above method, you not only force as many sperm towards the cervix, you also orient them along the perfect path to the eggs. If you have healthy sperm, the male sprinters will reach the egg first. If you are aiming for a girl, skip to the next chapter.

Following the rest period, it is okay to clean up the boss, but try to lie down for a nap. Enough of the sperm should have reached the deeper portions of the vagina after two hours. Do not urinate until then. Urine denatures sperm.

Lastly, remember to perform this recipe everyday for one week. You can throw away the "period" calendars and let go of the structured sexual encounters with your mate. Too much structure in sex will make it seem more of a chore than a party, and it should be the highlight of your day. Set a time for a date night or make it spontaneous. Get creative. By following the Dr. Blue Recipe once a day, you will be sure to cover her ovulation period, and then some. Make sure you keep things clean and wash-up after the rest periods so the boss stays healthy.

Think of the woman as a honey bear and you are trying to get the honey out, however in this scenario, you are trying to get as much honey *in* as possible. The Dr. Blue Recipe will give you the best chances of getting pregnant, and if the man's sperm are healthy, this method will produce a little boy.

# Persistent Little Girl

Life is full of surprises. Did you choose the right path at that fork in the road, or did you go left?

There is no way to sugar coat a bun without nuts. Yes, she is naturally sweet, loving, and kind hearted, but you will lose sleep. Long after the early days of her life, you will continue to lose sleep, and once you think she is safe, you will continue to lose sleep thinking about her. But she is worth every sleepless second!

Love her and she will love you back tenfold. Educate her and she will touch the lives of many. Protect her and she will never let you suffer. Do everything in your power to teach her wisdom, compassion, and confidence. She is impressionable and the decisions you make will influence her character. She is powerful, just like her mother, and she will set many traps. She needs both parents to grow properly. Do not let her become a trap to avoid.

Go back to that critical fork in the road during sexual intercourse. The woman has orgasmed from oral stimulation and the man has just reached the point of no return, seconds away from ejaculating. If you and your partner want a boy, you must plant your seeds deep into that broiling oven followed by the ever so important hand stand. But if you want a little girl, stay away from the hand stand and make those boy sperms run out of gas before getting to the finish line. Remember that girl sperms are endurance runners and the boys are sprinters. If you put them both close to the finish line, the sprinters will usually win. So you must back up the starting line to give the girls a better chance to finish first.

The Dr. Blue Recipe for a little girl:

Steps 1-5 are the same as a bun with nuts. Do not get lazy. The prep work is crucial!

1.  Once the woman has finished her menstrual cycle, wait 7 days and perform the following recipe once per day for the next 7 days.

2.  Preheat the oven. Begin by deeply kissing your woman. Gently touch and kiss every square inch of her amazing body. Make sure you turn on every nerve in her entire body and shut down the world around her in order to get the oven to broil.

3.  Once her body is properly preheated. Say hello to the little man in the boat. Make sure you tickle him with your tongue in a consistent, yet rapid motion. Stimulate that little man, commonly known as the clitoris, until he lets out a bolt of lightning throughout her entire body. Do not forget to give some love to the nipples.

4. Once your woman achieves an orgasm from oral stimulation by your tongue, quickly insert your penis into of her vagina. Get yourself to the verge of ejaculation as quickly as possible, but do not let it release.

5. In the seconds prior to ejaculation, pull your hips back and take a deep breath. Now transfer the energy inspired by that deep breath from your chest down to your core and out through your penis.

6. During the final push, do not extend your hips or squeeze your butt cheeks together. Instead, keep your hips in neutral while you go in as far as possible, and then pull back just slightly as you unleash your sperm. Let out a strong exhale as you contract your abdominals and pelvic floor muscles, squeezing every sperm out of your penis.

7. **THIS IS THE MOST IMPORTANT STEP**. Once all of your sperm have been unloaded, immediately lay her onto the bed into a horizontal position. No hand stand!

8. Let your woman rest while lying flat for 1-2 hours. Do not let her get up for anything. She can lift her head to drink

some water, but make sure she stays lying flat.

9.   Start thinking about baby girl names.


This recipe allows for a multitude of different positions to finish. If she wants to ride you until you orgasm, let her. If she wants you to do all the work, that's okay too.

The key to having a girl is to make the race to the egg long enough to allow the girl sperm to win. The hand stand is the clear advantage for the boy sperm. By avoiding the handstand, you make the race long enough for most of them to run out of gas.

A few tips to keep in mind: preheat the oven, hammer the little man in the boat until he shoots out lightning, and try to orgasm within 30 seconds of the woman's orgasm. This process is the key to life. You need a spark with the right conditions to create life.

For the man, it is not necessary for deep penetration. You actually do not want to be as deep as possible when you ejaculate.

Whether she is on top, missionary position, or any form of doggy style, place her on her back once you both orgasm.

Again, it is important not to urinate while the sperm are marinating inside the female.

This is all it takes to create a little girl. Repeat once a day for seven days straight. It may seem easier than the process of having a little boy, but beware. Little girls turn into big girls, and we all know big girls don't cry, but they do make grown men cry.

# Just Relax

Life is confusing, making a baby is not. Humans have been reproducing since day one and the most difficult part comes after the baby is delivered. It is frustrating for those who have tried many times to get pregnant with no success. We hear of those women who can get pregnant very easily, almost without any effort, while others pray until their hands bleed for a bun in the oven. There are some women who are not fit to care for children, yet they keep having babies. Others who may be highly qualified might never see the most precious word on that little stick doused with urine…PREGNANT.

The baby clichés are everywhere and the one *"it just isn't meant to be"* is tough for a couple to swallow after years of longing for a child of their own. The act of sex becomes routine and the romanticism goes out the window. Sex becomes more of a chore and less playful. Men become humiliated when they have to masturbate into a cup, stuck in a tiny medical office, afraid to touch anything and everything around them, yet hopeful that their count is adequate. Women, on the other hand, have to deal with the fact that they are an iceberg and most of their sexual physiology is underneath the surface, unable to be seen. They may feel helpless and become hopeless that they have no control over their body, repeatedly and voluntarily probed by their medical doctor with high hopes of solving their pregnancy questions. Some women have healthy eggs but they just will not stick. Some women are in their own heads too much and out think the power of the spark.

Whether you are trying to have a boy or girl, the key to life is adding a spark at the right time and in the right environment. Communication is sexy in a relationship and it not only builds trust, it also builds confidence in your partner. Talk about what makes you feel good. Go over the details of what turns you on and do not hold back. If you are truly serious about having a baby, make a sex plan. You both need to climax as close together as possible, and to make things tricky, a woman needs to climax through oral clitoral stimulation. This may make the man's job complicated, but discuss your plan. Keep a towel handy so you do not have to taste your own juices. If you need to begin with some slow penetration, that is okay. If you need to use some artificial lubricant to get things rolling, do it. Do not be embarrassed to tell your partner what you need in order to let go of the world around you and focus all of you energy into achieving an orgasm.

The first step is to relax the mind in order to properly prepare the body for the greatest miracle of all. Once her mind is in the right place and every inch of her body has been turned on, give the little man in the boat the business with your hammer until he cannot take anymore. When he lets out his bolt of lightning, put your dough into that oven and close the door. Then position her properly depending on which fork in the road you choose. Either road will take you on a wild adventure, and you will be tested, but most importantly, you will learn patience. Some days may be tougher than others, but you will learn that as you love your child, they will repay you exponentially.

Just remember to relax and do what nature has intended us to do.

And most importantly, make sure you don't call her an oven until she is actually pregnant.

www.ingramcontent.com/pod-product-compliance
Lightning Source LLC
Chambersburg PA
CBHW021337290326
41933CB00038B/942

* 9 7 8 0 6 9 2 5 8 1 3 0 8 *